FROM THE FAMILY DOCTOR TO THE CURRENT DISASTER OF CORPORATE HEALTH MAINTENANCE

How to Get Back to Real Patient Care!

THOMAS C. JONES;
BETSY M. CHALFIN

authorHOUSE®

AuthorHouse™ UK
1663 Liberty Drive
Bloomington, IN 47403 USA
www.authorhouse.co.uk
Phone: 0800.197.4150

Published by AuthorHouse 03/30/2016

ISBN: 978-1-5246-3122-2 (sc)
ISBN: 978-1-5246-3123-9 (hc)
ISBN: 978-1-5246-3121-5 (e)

Print information available on the last page.

This book is printed on acid-free paper.

CONTENTS

Problems and Potential Solutions for Today's Health Care System

One of the authors grew up with a wonderful family doctor—his father. In the early 1930s, that family doctor learned about how to care for his patients during four years of medical school. Most important, he learned how to empathize with his patients' needs and, then, how to do everything his knowledge permitted to ensure that their health benefited by putting his abilities into action.

This same author was so inspired by what he observed that he became a medical doctor and spent the rest of his life as a physician caring for patients, a teacher and a medical researcher.

This book recounts this author's observations and experiences toward the end of his medical career and ever since. His idealism was crushed as he observed many of his medical colleagues turn into spokesmen and spokeswomen for the pharmaceutical industry encouraging the use of expensive and unnecessary drugs and repetitive diagnostic tests. These same colleagues devolved into mere *personnel* of the for-profit hospital bureaucracies which affected their private practices as well. Ultimately, this devolution has consumed medical education and the teaching of medical ethics as well.

How did it happen? Was it an adverse event resulting from massive new technology? Was it a side effect of organizational restructuring? Was it induced by financial greed created by the pharmaceutical industry gone awry? Or was it the inevitable change created by a younger generation reinventing the idea of health care in response to a growing desire for youth and longevity? Most likely, it was similar to spontaneous combustion—an unforeseen and unfortunate result of the combination of all those factors.

There is no doubt that health care has evolved through many questionable practices over the centuries—from potions mixed by witch doctors to religious inhibitions placed on health care; to charlatans pushing imaginary cures—most often resulting in financial benefit or elevation in stature for those doing the "prescribing". But the process in place today has sunk to a level of subversion that appears to know no bounds.

This book is about the destruction of medical care as many of us knew it, and what we can and must do to correct the delivery of health care in the 21st century.

CHAPTER 1

Medicine from the 1930s to the 1970s

During the early decades of the 20th century, medical care underwent a great transformation. There were some incredible changes. For example, methods for diagnostic testing blossomed; vaccines were developed to prevent diseases like diphtheria, tetanus and polio; and therapies to cure severe infectious diseases appeared with the increased availability of penicillin and the development of new antibiotics.

Students attending medical school classes learned a great deal about these new advances, and they still learned about the primary role each of them had to play as the interlocutor of these advances between the emerging science and the patient.

This author keenly recalls several episodes as examples of the communication process when, as a medical student, he was permitted to observe the physician-patient interaction in his father's medical office. First, he noted that the waiting room was nicely decorated and quite comfortable. He learned later that many of the decorative paintings, lamps, and tapestries were gifts given by patients who could not afford to pay their medical bills in cash. He also learned that his father was always in trouble with the county medical society because he charged lower fees for his services to patients than the medical society advised. Dr. Jones would always say, "…I charge what my service is worth, not what someone else says my service is worth…"

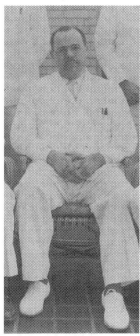
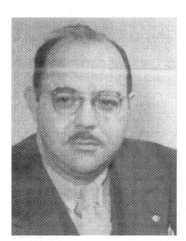

(Figs 1-1 and 1-2. The young Dr. John L. Jones in 1933
as a medical resident, then as a family doctor)

This author remembers one particular office visit with fondness.

Dr. John Jones was an obstetrician as well as a family doctor. One of his patients came to his office four weeks after the delivery of her baby and said, "Doctor, I know you said my husband and I should wait six weeks before having sex again, but my husband would like us to start sooner. What should I do?" In his most caring way Dr. Jones said, "Listen—I know your husband is a big strong guy. If he wants to have sex, I doubt if there is anything you or I should do to prevent it." The patient jumped up from her chair and said, "Oh thank you doctor!" That was a perfect example of family practice of health care.

This author also recalls that his father was always "on-call" and he also loved to cook. One Thanksgiving the whole family gathered together for dinner. Dr. Jones had the turkey roasting in the oven when he got a phone call from a patient whose baby decided it was time to be delivered. When he returned home later that night, after having delivered a healthy baby, he told us it was a bit difficult—he was not sure whether the baby was ready to deliver, or the turkey was ready to come out of the oven!

Also, in those days doctors had to combine the ingredients for patients' medications themselves. Dr. Jones would take great care in this process. He would study all aspects of the process and then worry about whether all would go well and his patient would improve. He gave advice to the worried-well, he gave injections to diabetics, he vaccinated children, and he treated ongoing infections. He was a family doctor.

CHAPTER 2

A Personal Recollection

When completely by chance I found myself in the world of medicine, it was a marvelous place. It was 1979. I had just returned to my birthplace—New York City. Master's Degree in hand, I embarked on a search for a job as a Special Education Teacher. Teaching jobs in my field were at a premium—mainstreaming of special education students was in its infancy and had significantly reduced the number of self-contained special education classrooms; as a result, cuts to special education budgets contributed to dwindling employment opportunities. I was sleeping on a friend's couch and, to ensure my ability to contribute my fair share during my job search, I signed on with a temporary personnel company—I was a fast typist and good speller so they quickly placed me as a "temp" in the Division of Infectious Diseases at Cornell University Medical College.

When I arrived for my first day of work, I learned that the doctor for whom I would be working was in India attending a medical conference. He had an active research laboratory; taught about infectious diseases and parasitology in the medical school; supervised the resident medical staff; saw hospital patients and private patients; and consulted on any number of obscure and complicated infectious diseases that I had never even heard of. In his absence, I was to begin setting up an organizational infrastructure for a soon-to-be-born Division of International Medicine.

Although I had always been interested in science and medicine, I never planned to pursue either as a career so it was quite unexpected when I found myself surrounded by smart, dedicated physicians and researchers. They were excited and enthusiastic about what they were doing—their goals of discoveries and cures were lofty. Information was enthusiastically shared in a collegial environment. There was a whole world of daily rounds, and grand rounds and morbidity and mortality conference every week; there were open symposia and discussions of basic research and laboratory techniques and successful and failed experiments. The dialogue was inclusive—professors, residents, nurses, medical students, researchers and laboratory technicians were all included. The attending physicians pored over the latest medical journals—certainly because they were interested but also because they lived in fear of a medical student or young resident asking them a question they might not know the answer to.

Speaking of medical students, they were a phenomenon. Bright, focused, energetic—they had great respect for the wisdom and experience of those they followed through the corridors on rounds, they were riveted during lectures, and always full of questions.

When something new was discovered in a particular laboratory, it belonged to the medical school. To the best of my knowledge, there were no patents on genetic material or research techniques; when a new bacteria was identified, it was named for a person—a patient, a doctor, a research technician. It was certainly not *owned* by any one person and certainly not by a giant pharmaceutical company or corporation. It may be hard to believe but, at that time, if a serious physician went to work for the pharmaceutical industry, he or she were considered to be a sell-out—a heretic—almost beneath contempt.

When the supervising physician I was yet to know—my boss—returned from India, I learned more about the new division he was creating. The Division of International Medicine was to be within the Department of Medicine—an off-shoot allied with, but separate from, the Division of Infectious Diseases.

With the dawn of global awareness brought vividly into our consciousness by television, the plight of millions living in under-developed countries that lacked adequate sanitation and food and water generated great interest among the medical community. There was a living laboratory ripe for study and discovery and, ultimately, greater attention, care and treatment. Everyone had heard of malaria and yellow fever— they had been rampant in the United States during the turn of the 20th century—but tropical diseases the average person knew nothing about were abundant— leishmaniasis, Chagas' disease, babesiosis, amebiasis.…

Research funded by philanthropy involving medical schools like Harvard, Johns Hopkins, Cornell University Medical College and others, had been underway for some years but on a relatively small scale. In a mere few years, the need for research into the lesser known diseases would sky-rocket with the advent of the HIV virus and the auto-immune deficiency syndrome (AIDS) because suddenly, immune suppression in our own patients opened the door to the invasion by these diseases right here in the United States.

As interest in infectious disease grew among medical students and residents, our division had an opportunity to join forces with a refugee relief organization that was providing medical services to the Cambodian refugees in a refugee camp located on the Thai-Cambodian border. With clarity about the urgency of the refugees' plight and great powers of persuasion, Ted Li, one of our medical residents, convinced Thomas Jones to support an effort to allow our residents, fourth year medical students, nurses, and attending physician staff to rotate through a field hospital in Khao I Dang refugee camp in Thailand. The potential learning and teaching opportunities for the students and staff were to prove nothing short of phenomenal—a once in a lifetime experience, not to mention the humanitarian contribution.

Amazingly, the administrations of the medical school and the hospital agreed to provide financial support in the form of continued salaries for the residents and faculty and they agreed that the Thailand experience would be considered an acceptable part of the elective curriculum. All of the administrative, travel and living expenses would be provided by the refugee relief organization. What evolved into a three year combined effort called the Cornell Thailand Program had an effect on all who participated in professional and personal experiences that carry over to today.

Would that kind of selfless enthusiasm for helping and learning among medical professionals and medical students be likely today? And would a medical school and a not-for-profit hospital be willing to pick up the tab? Woefully, I believe we know the answers to those questions.

Oh—I almost forgot—what *about* the money? And here begins the interesting tale of the devolution of the world of medicine as we now know it.

CHAPTER 3

The Emergence of the Pharmaceutical Industry and Medical Technology

The people developing and producing drugs and devices became very innovative in the later part of the 20th century. New antibiotics emerged, new diagnostic methods were developed, and new ways to define and treat diseases in a preventative way became apparent. These were the good news directions for this part of the scientific world, but then came the forces of evil. With so much success, there was suddenly needed better integration of effort, greater focus on the most profitable part of the developing science, marketing of new innovations, and an infrastructure to make sure it all worked for the benefit, not of patients, but of the investors in the pharmaceutical companies. This was to become an example of capitalism at its worst. But if this was not enough, further extensions were needed to ensure success.

These extensions included manipulation of the process of drug regulation and registration, advertisement of drugs in disingenuous ways to ensure maximum sales, and payments by pharmaceutical companies directly to physicians in order to ensure the widest distribution of the drugs and devices.

There are many examples of how the pharmaceutical industry has achieved amazing financial success. One particularly interesting and current example is the definition of potentially dangerous levels of cholesterol in the blood. The cholesterol levels were then correlated with cardiovascular events; the definition was then expanded to include the most borderline increased levels; then the definition was expanded to include people way outside of the age range that had been initially studied; then a class of drugs that could decrease the cholesterol levels, called statins, was developed. Finally the claim was—and continues to be—made that statins could reduce cholesterol levels, thereby reducing cardiovascular events, thus leading to prolonged life at any and all ages and, for just a small daily charge and a few more trips to your doctor to check for side effects, one could remain healthy by taking statin drugs for the entirety of one's life span.

We now know that the pharmaceutical companies who promoted these ideas have made billions of dollars but the role of statins has been recently reduced to a mixture of fantasy, ignorance of side effects, and false presentation. Statins can lower cholesterol but it turns out that this is a side effect of the drug, the main effects of which are to interfere with the mitochondrial metabolism of every cell in the body. In addition, lowering cholesterol does not alter the occurrence of cardiovascular diseases. Elevated cholesterol is simply a sign of metabolic disturbances which could possibly lead to vascular problems but the cholesterol level is not the cause.

The average cholesterol level in the population was 260, whereas the level at which the danger of vascular episodes was supposed to occur was stated to be 200— suddenly putting over 70% of the healthy population at risk. Lowering the blood cholesterol level did not alter a patient's underlying problem nor improve his or her life span, but it certainly put huge amounts of money in the coffers of the pharmaceutical companies.

A second example has been the new definition of hypertension and the need for lifelong anti-hypertension medication. A few years ago one was considered to have hypertension with a blood pressure of 150/100; then this number was reduced to 140/90. On what basis was this change made? We may not know why the change was made but we do know that it resulted in many more drugs being sold to more people.

A third example is the new definition of type 2 diabetes—a number applied to the fasting blood sugar allowed a whole population of primarily overweight people to start taking anti-diabetic drugs.

Further examples include the revised definitions of Parkinson's disease and Alzheimer's disease coinciding with pharmaceutical companies developing drugs for life-long treatment of these diseases. The frequency among the aging population increased from a few hundred thousand people to tens of millions. The claim has been made that because of longer survival ages, these diseases emerge. But when one analyzes the mathematics of such claims one will see that these diseases, which can only be diagnosed by observing patterns of clinical symptoms, have increased because of a change in definitions. These definitions were reinterpreted by the pharmaceutical companies making the new drugs and have been applied by the physicians that benefit from the financial support provided to them by the pharma companies, government Medicare and Medicaid, private insurance companies and increased patient visits required to monitor the effects of the drugs being prescribed.

Another problem in the process of drug and medical device development has been the questionable government oversight system. The Federal Drug Administration (FDA) has been a powerful force in the regulation of medicines and medical devices in the United States for over 50 years. During the past few decades, FDA policies have begun to be mirrored in many other parts of the world, most notably in Europe.

The power of the FDA and its expanding influence derived from several factors but, most important, from the desire of citizens to feel secure that a prescription medicine or an over-the-counter (OTC) drug has been properly tested and is safe for use. Due to a number of subtle mis-labeling practices by the FDA, however, its role has expanded significantly, and at tremendous cost, to include the entire process of regulating health care.

The FDA promotes itself as a government agency established to "protect the public" but, using that definition, it has become a micromanager of all aspects of health care in our society. If each person knew what they had given up in the process of this evolution from drug safety to total drug control, we are certain there would be a request to take some of their own decision-making power back. Citizens should ask for a marked reduction in the power of the FDA and for a return to its role as a safety monitor rather than a drug controller.

High administrative costs, blunting drug development, and delays in drug and medical device availability have been well detailed in the book, *Hazardous to Our Health? FDA Regulation of Health Care Products* edited by Robert Higgs. Higgs describes that the FDA is not a body to ensure drug safety, but rather a law-enforcement and political body that has the goal to regulate, supervise, and partly determine the development, manufacture, advertising, and availability of all drugs.

Just over the past 10 years, the cost of drug development has increased up to ten-fold; as a result of the processes in place, delays in drug availability have increased two- to three-fold. This is only the tip of the iceberg, resulting from misguided trust in an agency originally established to supervise drug and device safety. There are numerous examples of how the change in operation of the FDA over the years has denied the public, including elders, numerous medications. Due to a number of bureaucratic obstacles, some people have had to wait for years to obtain a drug shown to be both effective and safe and widely used in other countries. Some drugs can only be obtained by going to Canada, which may be illegal, or by shopping on the internet.

The FDA has clearly misrepresented itself as an organization that ensures the safety of medicines and devices; in reality, the FDA is blocking and delaying creative drug development, increasing health care costs, and using government funds to pay the salaries of their army of statisticians, micromanagers and bureaucrats. The agency involves itself in the composition of hospital clinical review boards, in the design of the clinical investigation process, and in manipulating the scientific direction of pharmaceutical research. This last point was made clear when a former FDA head told top executives of pharmaceutical companies to begin research on agents to inhibit the HIV virus or to not bother bringing any drug for approval to the FDA. We may happen to share an enthusiasm for HIV research, but we cannot support the role of the FDA as a threatening force in the process. The FDA was doing the wrong thing under the wrong label.

Of course, regulatory agencies do not create deceptive practices alone. There is evidence that pharmaceutical companies and government finance offices participate as well, particularly in Europe. An example of pharmaceutical company participation putting up barriers to drug approval was seen recently in the new European Union rules regarding clinical trials necessary to register a drug already registered in one formulation—for example, a topical agent being available in a liquid solution instead of a cream.

Many years ago, a logical and inexpensive approach was required simply to prove that a new formulation did not alter tolerability, stability, or absorption of a drug. Since the active drug was already tested and registered, if no chemical alteration was demonstrated then the new formulation was registered. Now, major and costly drug development is required, as if a new formulation contains some new agent. This change requires action by a pharmaceutical company that costs anywhere from $500,000 to $10,000,000.

Surprisingly the pharmaceutical companies supported this change, but why? This is a step in what used to be called "life-cycle management" of a drug. The pharmaceutical company's corporate financial and legal officers realized there was a far greater danger to their company than the added cost of a new study. That greater danger was future competition from companies who could make generic copies of their drug after the patent expired. The new rule makes it very expensive for a generic company to get into the game. So, who pays for this added cost? The public pays—fewer formulations of drugs are available and the potential reduction in drug costs is limited.

By misrepresenting its activities, the FDA has duped the public into thinking that tax dollars are being used to protect them when, in fact, the FDA and other regulatory agencies have been denying the public potential life-saving medications marketed in a timely manner thereby resulting in increased health care costs. The approach taken by the regulatory agencies has had far reaching effects on the entire structure of the pharmaceutical industry. The new structure has led to the replacement of innovation with lots of paper, individual initiative with corporate regulatory-driven dictates, and personal responsibility with collective supervision.

There have also been impressive advances in medical technology. This means that techniques became available to intervene in all aspects of health care by the use of primarily surgical procedures to replace arteries in the heart, to replace hips, to do diagnostic scans of the entire body looking for potential problems, and to prolong life for the injured and elderly in intensive care units. This technology has resulted in many advantages but the resulting financial windfall to hospitals and health care organizations requires further evaluation.

CHAPTER 4

The Science of Medicine
Has Been Corrupted

As a physician, it has been difficult for one of the authors of this book to admit that the science he studied and believed in could be the source of a form of corruption never anticipated. Here are the data that confirm that fact.

The most important basis of proper medical practice has always been *what and where are the facts*? That all important foundation is where the problem begins. The facts for all decisions made by doctors today have been so altered that one must wonder how it is possible to perform the important task of relating their patient to the scientific evidence.

There are so many places where a doctor must rely on facts, let us consider a few examples.

1) What are the statistics at the basis of a scientific recommendation?

2) Can clinical trials of a new drug or procedure be relied upon? In other words, were the data reported in a reliable manner?

3) Was a minor alteration in health care benefit or harm described as a major breakthrough or disaster by academic and journalistic magnification? 4) When did the marketing of a new drug or technique become more important than the actual innovation of the product?

4) When did a physician's careful assessment of medical facts become influenced by the potential for financial gain if he or she simply accepted the information provided?

We will explore how, when and where the answers to these questions became so complex that patient care and the relationship between a physician and his patient began to suffer.

- Statistics

One of the most surprising facts is that the numbers all doctors have been taught to rely on for decision-making have been altered to such an extent that they must now be viewed as totally unreliable. These numbers, after a bit of manipulation, are referred to as statistics.

The problem is that each time we look at a list of data, we are urged to simplify the list by adding things together; then by placing percentages on the information; then by deciding, based on artificial constructs, whether anything significant has occurred.

An example of this problem was provided by Dr. Ben Goldacre in his book, *Bad Science*. He reported that those who had high blood cholesterol were 50% more likely to have a heart attack than those with normal cholesterol levels. Goldacre then pointed out that we should have looked at the "actual numbers", not the artificial percentage. The actual numbers show that 4 of 100 people with normal cholesterol have a heart attack, whereas 6 of 100 people with high cholesterol will have a heart attack. One immediately sees that this difference of 2% (4 to 6 people of 100) cannot possibly be a reason to place thousands of people on a drug to lower cholesterol (with the well-recorded side effects of the drug). But this 2% difference was placed in the literature as a 50% increase—ie. an increase from 4 people to 6 people). The false statistics became the justification for a lie that took decades to correct.

Another example of the use of false statistics is the reliance on the .05 p value to determine significant differences between two populations of numbers—a totally manufactured value. The effects of a substance administered to one group were compared to those in a group who received no drug (the placebo group). How did such an artificial number (.05) become the key to the marketing of a new drug?

Another example has been to compare two groups that are both considered to have received active compounds by use of "confidence limits". It has become very clear that the one thing to do is to place no confidence in confidence limits.

Statistical analysis has become a self-serving game played by people who are hired as *statisticians*. Unfortunately, statisticians are generally hired to do their jobs by the people that have already decided what the results need to be. We will discuss later the issue of hiding data that does not conform to the desired answers but, for now, be aware of the problem of bad statistics.

- ## False reporting of clinical trials data

In his book *Bad* Pharma, also written by Ben Goldacre, he clearly makes the point that *all* of the clinical trials carried out on a new chemical entity or a new procedure are not reported—only the positive ones are. This reporting failure is well known to the pharmaceutical industry, to most academic physicians, and to the regulatory agencies—but it goes on almost totally uncontrolled. This occurs partly because many journals and the press do not like to report negative findings because no one wants to read such reports. So, even if a conscientious drug developer wants to publish all of the observations made, he cannot get the findings published.

The Journal of Negative Results in Biomedicine is available for those in research to publish their negative findings. Rather than submit their negative observations for publication, in most cases it has become more convenient for the drug developer to have a special bottom drawer in which to file negative observations to be referred to at a future time rather than submit them for publication. So, the data are not really hidden—they are just filed in a separate place.

- ## Have journalists done their jobs?

The answer to that question is obvious. Journalists have done what they always do—present the best story about what is happening that they can. There is little doubt that the corporate world is very aware that only the best and most exciting news about any drug or medical appliance or treatment is what gets reported. So are the journalists responsible for this mess?

We, the authors of this book, believe that they share in the responsibility. They not only fail to properly report all of the information available but, along with doctors, CEOs, and the federal government, they receive income despite their incomplete reportage. In addition, the journals that are supposed to provide the best up-to-date information benefit from advertising paid for by the very companies they are supposed to be impartially evaluating. The free exchange of information has been a major casualty in the current process of maintaining the status quo of health care provided in the United States.

Dr. Goldacre is a British physician working in the United Kingdom. He addresses the issues that affect the US and the medical system globally but the problems he addresses, despite their importance, are only a small part of the disaster of health care in the United States.

For just one example, it is illegal in the United Kingdom to publish articles that support specific drugs in the UK press. In contrast, in the US the types of articles that lead patients to consider all sorts of false claims are perfectly legal. This must stop if we are to protect society from quackery.

- When did marketing become the hallmark of a great pharmaceutical company?

Sometime several decades ago the research and development of innovative pharmaceutical products turned from an innovative health care process into a market driven investor protective process. The process is such that it has recently been reported that pharmaceutical companies now spend 85% of their income on marketing and human resources, and only 15% on the actually finding and developing new medical care products.

One might say that providing health care has always involved making money for the provider, but, during the time of my father's family medical practice, it never occurred to anyone that making money was his motivation. Something very damaging has happened in the past few decades that must be investigated and accurately reported.

- When did a physician's evaluation of the facts become so influenced by financial gain?

There is little doubt that the creation of the Health Maintenance Organization (HMO) has played a major role in the way medicine is currently practiced in the US. The family doctor has disappeared, the patient advocate has disappeared, and the selfless patient-directed medical provider has disappeared. This person who encompassed all three roles has been replaced by an organization of corporate executive officers, managers, and financial efficiency experts. One cannot really blame the doctors—they have essentially been pawns in a very lucrative chess game. Many of these doctors did not realize the extent to which their performance would be monitored by the number of patients they saw and the number of prescriptions they wrote. If a certain threshold was not maintained, likely he would be replaced by a more efficient member of the medical profession.

This author feels certain that, faced with such a contract, he would never have signed on—but who can be sure? This book represents an attempt to defend the unfortunate doctor who tried to stand up against such pressure.

CHAPTER 5

The Sub-Speciality Boom

In the United States a process of patient care began to emerge such that the family doctor was no longer in charge of his or her patient's care, but instead became the first step in a complex network of referrals. The family doctor was now the *primary physician*.

The primary, or "first line" physician, was there simply to offer a suggestion of a possible medical problem. Then, with appropriate or inappropriate reimbursement, the patient is given a referral to the next level sub-specialist. This change in the health care network made it very attractive for a young physician-in-training to aspire to qualify as that sub-specialist.

The subspecialist has the expertise, the specialized equipment, and the motivation that justifies charging the patient far more than the primary care physician can.

Another factor that might not have required such consideration in earlier times was that the amount of debt incurred by the combined cost of a college education and medical school would grow to nearly $500,000. A new physician needed greater remuneration to pay off debt; another motivation to seek sub-specialist status.

To be fair, this emerging trend was not all about money; it was also about having the most up-to-date equipment so the best possible medical assessment could be made. The cardiology specialist now had access to imaging equipment and cardio-invasive tools in addition to the X-ray and the electrocardiograph. The gastroenterologist had more sophisticated equipment to perform endoscopy and colonoscopy along with access to new imaging procedures and space-age surgical techniques. All of this also required trained technical staff and a place to perform special procedures. Ambulatory care and surgi-centers were on the horizon. Now that the imaging equipment was available to carry out tests that were not considered vital at an earlier time, gynecologists decided that it was important to measure bone density and new pharmaceuticals allowed pre and post menopausal treatment and more follow-up visits. Why would any physician want to simply talk with a patient and think about the best care and treatment once all of these special (and expensive) tools were available! One would be crazy to remain in the position of a primary care physician with all of this incredible technology going on in the sub-specialty fields.

The appearance of the sub-specialist also led the primary care physician to seek an organizational network to insure he or she was getting a fair share of the heath care lucre. This was a sufficiently complex structure that justified a new administrative bureaucracy including corporate organizers and financial officers to orchestrate the process. Hence, the impetus for the creation of a Health Maintenance Organization—the HMO—was born.

CHAPTER 6

The Health Maintenance Organization

One of the most significant developments in the history of health care in the United States has been the emergence of Health Maintenance Organizations—the HMO.

It appears that physicians did not have sufficient managerial skills so someone else had to take on the task of managing their medical practices. It is probably true that doctors were not very good managers but what emerged to make up for their short comings has been a nightmare for patient care.

In 1973, The Health Maintenance Organization Act amended the previous Public Health Service Act of 1944. This legislation effectively transformed the way health benefits were to be managed in America and around the world. Under the current legal code, an HMO is defined as a public or private entity that meets two specific requirements: 1) it provides basic and supplemental health services to its members; and 2) it is organized and operated in accordance with state-approval. In essence, an HMO is an organization created to provide equal access to health care services in exchange for members agreeing to specific terms. Generally, this is an agreement that requires physicians to participate within a covered network of providers who have pre-negotiated itemized costs for services, while still retaining quality of care.

Despite good intentions, most HMOs gradually morphed into health care bureaucracies that charge excessive fees for health maintenance of questionable quality; they pay considerable salaries to their executive staff; they control the income of the participating physicians; and overall have greatly increased the total cost of health care in the United States. This has, in fact, become a disaster on many levels.

Perhaps the worst part of the development of HMOs is that it reduced the role of the family doctor—now the primary care physician—to one who enters data into a laptop computer, reviews laboratory reports, and passes the patient up the ladder. The HMO structure became so successful that no family doctor could possibly compete. Rather than starve, the family doctor joined on to the company. Now as the primary care doctor, their job was to recruit and maintain new patients; ensure that the patient received long-term medical treatment; and at the end of the patient's life to recommend intense, expensive, hospital-based care rather than staying at home with an in-home care giver or loving family member. If the doctor failed to toe the line—in other words, not maintain a roster of follow-up visits, not refer enough patients for imaging and repetitive tests, or spent too much time with patients—he or she was declared incompetent and their employment terminated.

The process of managing health care in the United States might be a fascinating evolutionary study if the managed care experiment had not been so successful and so devastating for patients, physicians and even to financial investors. In light of the uncertainties governing the socioeconomic structure in the United States, it is difficult to predict what the ultimate outcome will be.

How is it that people with reasonable intellect in a democratic health care-conscious society have allowed such a system to emerge?

The major problem with the original system was that it was inefficient, according to Dr. Hazzard in a recent article, and inefficiency resulted in obstacles to access of health care.

We will confirm that the system was not very efficient. Work hours were long, house calls were frequent, and the effort to carry out academic research alongside of patient care was not always handled effectively. Care could have been improved by including medical planners to observe, assess and streamline procedures and, in retrospect, it is a mistake that this was not done. Instead, managed care became an experiment in financial restructuring—not in efficient health care delivery.

As reviewed by Hall and Berenson, managed care emerged without first developing associated ethical standards in the delivery of health care. Managed care allowed the substitution of a commercial system for the physician's guardian role in health care.

The results have been unfortunate. There are many people who have no access to health care at all. Physicians are trying to rebalance their humanitarianism, their medical ethics, their independence, their very existence within this system. It seems apparent that so much restructuring has occurred and the current system is so complicated, it is difficult to see how significant changes can be designed and implemented.

How did it happen that health care—a basically humanitarian process with its core in the doctor-patient relationship—with its demanding educational preparation and its social focus on all aspects of birth, life, fear, pain and death became a primarily commercial activity?

As summarized in another context by Dr. Barondess, health care has followed totally incorrect paths before. We can point to a few key elements which may have led to the present managed care industry in the United States.

First, in many ways managed care is a product of the technological revolution. There are two major issues that result from the availability of new technology. The first, described in a book review by Dr. Relman, is that the expense and the expectations regarding new technology has led to a gap between funds available for health care delivery and patient demands. The new technology caused the problem but then the economic sector, not the medical-ethical sector, was sought to solve the problem.

The second issue is that, in the past, the practice of medicine placed the physician as a comforter partly because there was no special technology to utilize to intervene in the illness of his patients.

We must ask the question, therefore, how do we ensure that the most up-to-date technology is made available to each patient and not lose the humanitarian role of the physician at the same time? The answer requires that we consider whether technology and humanity are mutually exclusive. The answer is no.

Physicians must be taught how to evaluate the appropriate technology for each patient (that is, to apply ethical considerations not economic considerations), and then they must learn how to refer each patient in the most thoughtful way to those who can deliver the new technology (that is, be a wise comforter). This is a process of medical education not bureaucratic management. We must then ensure that the physician at each level of the patient's care is appropriately reimbursed for his actions. This is a civil-social process not bureaucratic management.   The way new technology affected patient care was ignored at the start of this revolution. Patients saw their physician becoming more and more distant. Their physician was then replaced by a new and very different kind of primary care physician. At the same time, the cost of their care dramatically increased. Finally, the medical system as the patient once knew it was totally replaced by a managed commercial system.

In retrospect, the mistakes made in the 1970s were not only to underestimate the impact of the cost of new technology on the system but also not to supplement the technologist, or the specialist, with another layer of care closer to the patient. As described by Davidoff, we all went in the wrong direction toward commercialism rather than toward a humanitarian use of new technology.

One of the dreams of those who supported managed health care was that by implementing efficient management, the inadequate distribution of health care in the United States would be solved. On the surface, this thinking is as reasonable as placing another layer of health care providers when technology is too complex. It was thought that if health care was not available to all, it was due to inefficiency in the delivery system—therefore, fix the delivery system.

Unfortunately we have learned that altering the delivery system does not necessarily ensure broader access to that health care system. In the present managed care system, poor distribution of care persists but the economics of the system places money in different pockets.

The message to those in other countries is that one cannot solve poor distribution of health care by bringing in market driven administrators and economists. Instead, it must be done by designing a comprehensive system for distribution of resources in a manner that assures the availability of preventive medical care, nutrition and intervention health care for all. This would necessarily be a large industry combining taxation, insurance, and efficient decision making. Health care planners would have to be involved, along with political facilitators and physicians, but the goal would have to be humanitarian-oriented health care not financial profit. The absence of the humanitarian oriented component is the major failing of the managed care experiment in the United States.

One of the reasons the HMO experiment was done in the United States was because a basic enthusiasm for the market place as a social balance existed. An underlying current of opinion suggested that good people deserve things and they do not require a support system; bad people do not deserve things and they are socially costly; and market forces would decide all potential imbalances in the middle.

The approach to managed care in the US will be discussed for a long time, but it is our hope that the major benefit of the experiment will be to turn a spotlight on the fallacy of the direction taken. Market forces will never have as a goal the kind of humanitarian effort needed to ensure the health care of a society. As recently stated, those forces are not likely able to save the market let alone the well-being of individuals in a society. Andrulis recently emphasized that appropriate plans for access to medical care must focus on socioeconomic disparities first—the present system has not followed this course.

One must ask where the medical leadership in the United States was while this transformation was taking place. Medical practice in the US has been guided by the major physicians organization, The American Medical Association (AMA). This organization has done many good things including serving as a major source of information exchange; it has been a bridge between standards of care provided by physicians and political, legal, para-professional organizations and, most of all, an organization that has spoken out in favor of the established system of providing health care. But unfortunately, during the restructuring process the AMA failed to provide the needed perspective of the guardian of health. This was due partly to cultural fears that led to rejection of the sweeping change in approach to health care proposed by the US administration in 1994, but also because of the AMA's traditional role as a physicians' union.

It is true that ethical issues related to new plans for a health care system were discussed in 1994, but recommendations arising from these discussions were placed on the side-line. Had the AMA been willing to publically acknowledge the problems of the distribution of fees, the obstacles that prevent access to health care, the lack of clarity about how and when hospital beds and new technologies should be used and, perhaps most important, the lack of focus on the importance of preventive health care, it may have been better able to contribute as a respected component of the solution.

Spokesmen within the AMA have continued to try to reshape the course of events. The American College of Physicians has also called on all physicians to become leaders in a movement to achieve universal access to health care but, according to all indications, these activities are too little and far too late.

It would have been difficult to imagine as recently as a few years ago that a significant symptom of the disaster of US health care would be that many physicians went bankrupt because the managed care facilities for which they worked made serious financial mistakes. Little has been done to put in place the oversight necessary to ameliorate this ongoing problem.

CHAPTER 7

Hospitals—For-profit Corporations; No Longer Non-profit Community-based Care Centers

One of the most unfortunate changes in the US health care system has been the gradual disappearance of the community hospital. Community-based hospitals were tax-exempt non-profit institutions largely supported with county and state funds ear-marked for health care and by private charitable contributions. Once gone, for-profit hospitals have taken their place. These hospitals are usually part of a larger holding company run according to a business model and run by Corporate Executive Officers.

This change in the hospital paradigm might not have proved so disastrous had the newly entrenched CEOs not made their primary task the creation of profit for those who were running the holding companies of which the hospital was a part. To accomplish this task a process often referred to as re-engineering was undertaken. Re-engineering focused on profit-making activities that were reimbursed by government programs like Medicare and Medicaid and by private insurance companies. An ever increasing number of expensive medical tests; imaging; scanning; and special procedures like arteriography and cardiac catheterization—all requiring special facilities and specialized care— were prescribed. Rather than refer patients to outside independent facilities, hospitals began opening their own imaging centers and ambulatory care facilities. These frequent, redundant and often unnecessary procedures have contributed considerably to the soaring cost of medical care. This routine escalates to the point of end-of-life care when it is now considered state-of-the-art to sequester elder patients in intensive care units where extraordinary measures are often taken in order to prolong life with no thought of quality of life, despite the fact that most of these patients would prefer to be at home in peaceful familiar surroundings.

A man a bit over 85 years old was diagnosed as having cancer of the prostate. A well-respected specialist in an independent medical practice suggested that treatment would likely not be helpful and that at his advanced age the treatment was worse than the disease.

In contrast, the man's primary Medicare supported HMO doctor urged an aggressive approach in the form of 27 radiation treatments with each treatment costing Medicare $1,100. Based on his long established relationship with his primary physician he agreed to the treatment plan. After nine radiation treatments he could not tolerate any more and ceased treatment. The treatment left him incontinent. A few years later, now dying of old age, he let himself be talked into a lung biopsy to see if the cancer "had spread" by his same for-profit HMO doctor who told him the biopsy would be no more uncomfortable than a "mosquito bite." Following the biopsy, he ended up in the Intensive Care Unit; $170,000 later he was in agony, had a serious infection, and died miserably several months later.

Family members have often asked, "Why should 90% of our medical care dollars be spent during the last six months of our lives and why should elders be tortured with treatments that are worse than their diseases?" Why spend one's last months in a hospital when one could have around-the-clock treatment at home at much less expense? Why?"

In conjunction with the new paradigm of hospital care, a system of billing practices were put in place that are truly unique in the history of medicine. It appears that the government programs of Medicare and

Medicaid were willing to pay only 20% of the growing cost for patients in the hospital on a diminishing scale with the greatest reimbursement paid for the first day of hospitalization. In response, the hospital CEOs established a system that automatically charged any patient being paid for by such means about five times the actual cost. If one received such a bill and was willing to pay by cash or credit card, the bill was reduced to 20%! Of course this decision by the hospitals was made so they could be certain they would recover the full amount of their actual expenses, not just 20%.

So why did the federal government come up with this plan? There is only one logical reason—someone was aware that there was a five-fold over-billing by the hospitals. Maybe we should find out what has really been going on with hospital billing then begin a class action suit against hospitals for fiscal negligence to recover the billions of dollars that patients have been inappropriately billed for. Perhaps that will be the only way to get the numbers right going forward.

CHAPTER 8

Doctors Must Choose Between Profit or Pro-patient Care—Profit Wins

The most painful part of this story is that physicians really do like to help their patients, and they like to view themselves as care givers to society. It appears that they have been put in an untenable position. On one hand, physicians could do what the old family doctor did and accept a small fee for guiding their patient through the maze of tests and treatments; or they could look at their life style and their personal and family expenses, and accept payments and follow directions meted out by the pharmaceutical companies or the CEOs of the HMOs. This is certainly a tough choice for any conscientious doctor to make.

CHAPTER 9

Can the Unintended Decline of Patient Care be Reversed?

The answer to that question of whether or not the decline of patient care can be reversed is, Yes it can! The "how" answer is the one we address in this chapter of our book.

First, we must all think about how the current state of medical care came about during the past 30 to 40 years. Several significant things that affected the original system of medical care occurred:

1) The pharmaceutical industry turned from a primarily scientific structure to a regulated marketing and investor- oriented structure;

2) The technologic basis of medicine changed in that new technologies in diagnosis and patient care became much more complex and expensive;

3) Health care funding became confused and inefficient at all levels of government and in the insurance industry;

4) University and medical school education became much more expensive, so that young doctors were heavily in debt at the time they graduated; and

5) The common belief emerged that business experts, not medical doctors, could run the complex process of patient care—hence, the HMO.

There are a number of steps that must be taken to correct the present situation. First, we must bring together all of those who really believe that patient care is an absolute right of every person. Second, we must make sure that the solution to this problem uses a social justice approach rather than an approach which is a capitalistic reinvention of society.

We have heard that young people who want to be physicians are being driven into sub-specialty careers because the task of the primary care physician is so unclear or has been down-graded to merely a referral position. This must change. We must re-establish the primary care giver as the most important one in our society. If we cannot do that by employing financial incentives then we must identify a different set of rewards for those who, like my father, are willing to sacrifice almost anything to ensure the best outcomes for their patients and their families.

Of course one way to ensure the future of the primary care physician in our society is to make certain that any graduate of a medical or nursing school is not saddled with enormous education debts; they must be assured of a reasonable income provided, perhaps, by federal or state funding; and that they have a choice in the method they want to use to implement their skills and deliver the quality care they learned about during medical their education. These straight-forward steps would bring about a dramatic change in the present direction of health care—perhaps too dramatic for the United States citizenry.

Other countries in the world, particularly those in Scandinavia, put straight-forward systems of health care for all in place many years ago and they have societies that continue to put social responsibility to their communities above individual profit margins and capital gain. Is such a socially responsible community still possible in the United States? Perhaps not—but the authors of this book hope so.

CHAPTER 10

Pharmaceutical Advertising and the Need for Regulation

We have all been bombarded by pharmaceutical advertising for years. Sadly, much of this advertising is so effective that it drives patients to demand that their physicians write prescriptions for specific drugs, despite the fact that the particular drug may or may not be appropriate for them or that the same drug components are available in a less expensive generic version.

One of the reasons for all of this advertising is that, about 20 years ago, the government restricted pharmaceutical companies from sending their sales people to medical schools and hospitals armed with gifts like medical equipment and baseball tickets and certificates for high end restaurant meals so they might gain entrée to pitch their newest product to the medical students and residents who were not yet well-acquainted with many of the pharmaceuticals. In addition, the pharmaceutical companies would recruit often well-known physicians to pitch products for them by offering them honoraria or trips to exotic locales. Since they could no longer use their promotional budgets to directly persuade physicians to prescribe their products, they reallocated those promotional dollars to the air waves and to a more easily persuaded public.

The current formula used in advertising essentially turns scientific advances into marketing tools for prescription drugs and medical appliances that flaunt minor achievements as if they were the ultimate cure for one disease or another.

We have observed this advertising in various media platforms. In addition to television advertising that utilizes attractive models who appear totally healthy despite whatever ailment they claim to have had before taking the miracle drug, there is the glitzy magazine advertising. Usually, the advertisement consists of two pages—the first is a full color page with a photo or company banner accompanied by a list of the great things the drug does, followed by a second page of microscopic fine print that, if read carefully, describes so many side effects—including death—to protect them from liability if anyone who dares take the drug falls seriously ill or dies.

Companies get away with grandiose claims despite the efforts of the Federal Trade Commission which is responsible for protecting consumers from deceptive marketing practices. Clever marketers create advertisements that *imply* cures without directly claiming that their product cures a particular condition or illness. They are masters at creating impressions with images of happy people or healthy children playing with cute puppies while employing terminology like "live longer" or "boosts immunity" –claims that cannot be quantified one way or the other. In particular, the health concerns of the elder population are fodder for exaggerated claims for products like "memory boosting" drugs.

Some of the pharmaceutical claims are so implausible that it is truly surprising that magazines are willing to publish them.

I wrote a letter and challenged the advertising policy of a journal I received and I was told, in writing, that the journal was complying with all legal requirements regarding advertisements. Needless to say, I cancelled my subscription. It continues to baffle me that such advertising is illegal in the United Kingdom but not in the United States? Why are citizens in the United States not afforded the same protection from deceptive television and magazine advertising as those in other countries—much as we are protected from charlatans hawking snake oil cures? It seems obvious that the protection of the public health requires that truth in advertising rules must be restored or rewritten.

Another aspect of pharmaceutical advertising is that academic physicians and journalists are paid to write articles supporting the drugs that the pharmaceutical companies are touting. Some of these articles are written by the company and the physician simply allows his or her name to be attached. At this time there is no requirement that such payments or in-kind remuneration be clearly disclosed.

The only way to put an end to this blatant form of persuasion is to make it illegal for the pharmaceutical industry to advertise products or to make unsubstantiated claims about their achievements.

CHAPTER 11

Carefully Defining Diseases Including Patients Age Range and Diagnostic Limits

One of the most complex problems in the process of patient care is identifying when a patient must be recognized as having a specific disease. There is a now famous quote from Aldous Huxley: "If you believe you are healthy, you need more diagnostic testing."

The identification and diagnosis of a specific disease is often made based on a collection of signs and symptoms that the physician must analyze in order to form a clinical judgment. Regrettably, this process has been complicated by the efforts of the pharmaceutical industry to create diagnoses by applying artificial numbers or manipulating statistics thereby increasing the number of prescriptions being written.

One early example of this numeric manipulation was the confusing of rheumatoid arthritis and relevant drug treatments, with osteoarthritis (a misnomer as it is really an arthropathy, not an arthritis). This confusion allowed drugs used to control inflammation to be used on a disease process (osetoarthropathy) that actually required more inflammation for healing, not less. Another example is the change in the definitions of hypertension, of hypercholesterolemia, and of type 2 diabetes by simply lowering the levels to achieve the definition. The definition of type 2 diabetes is particularly interesting because the definition applies particularly to obese adults who should lose weight but decide to ask their doctor what they should do. The doctor tells the patient that he or she must have regular medical checkups, test their blood sugar level several times each day, and take a pill regularly to reduce their high blood sugar level.

A friend of mine followed this advice but noted that, while taking the prescribed medication, her blood sugar levels were too low. The doctor's advice regarding this problem: "Just eat more when the blood sugar level recorded is too low!"

Most recently, the terms Parkinson's Disease and Alzheimer's Disease have been redefined such that the number of patients administered prescription drugs has expanded to the millions.

In 1980, it was reported that there were 1 million Americans with Parkinson's disease and 50,000 new cases of Parkinson's diagnosed each year. By 2010, the number of cases had risen to 15 million with 60,000 new cases each year. The mathematics of this increase cannot be due to increased numbers of aged people— it can only be due to a change in the criteria used to make a clinical diagnosis. In addition, Parkinson's disease rose to the second most commonly diagnosed neurologic illness.

Parkinson's is a disease associated with a decrease in dopamine levels in the brain occurring primarily between ages 50 and 70 (but now identified in those under age 50 and over 80 years of age). The disease is primarily observed as "tremors while at rest" but this criteria is being amended to include all sorts of potential early signs. Parkinson's had to be distinguished from *essential tremor* which was previously the much more common illness in the aged population. Essential tremor is defined as "a tremor that occurs when one begins to move a group of muscles". The distinction had to be made by the physician using clinical criteria—in other words there was no associated marker or medical test to confirm or reject the clinical diagnosis.

Of course once the diagnosis of Parkinson's disease is made a patient must receive life-long medical follow-up visits, daily medication, frequent blood tests to monitor potential side effects of the new drugs, and ongoing payments directly to the physician or health maintenance organization from an insurance company.

First on the list of the most common neurologic illnesses is Alzheimer's disease that was first described by Alois Alzheimer in Germany in 1906. Alzheimer's disease was much less common than senile dementia, vascular brain damage, or simple memory loss just a few decades ago. The rarity was partly due to the fact that it could only be diagnosed by the appearance of the brain at autopsy. However, new interest in early diagnosis and therapy has increased the number of cases in the United States to 4 to 5 million in 2000, with an estimated increase to 13 million by 2050.

In recent years, numerous medications have been developed in an attempt to slow the progress of mental deterioration, thus encouraging patients and health care providers to make a diagnosis as early as possible.

But remember, the diagnosis is made primarily by excluding other diseases with similar symptom patterns. How can a health care provider be objective given the financial incentive to make a diagnosis and commence treatment and the potential good will of the patient who thinks a new remedy may be available? Circumstances like these create a perfect setting for enthusiastic over-diagnosis.

CHAPTER 12

Removing For-profit Health Maintenance Organizations

It should be easy to get rid of the health maintenance organizations (HMOs) that make exorbitant profits from the health care industry despite the fact that the administrators who garner most of the income actually provide no direct care to patients. The simple solution is to remove the profit-making component from the organization. Once profit is no longer the organizational goal, the CEOs of the HMOs and those who invest in these organizations would vanish. Of course there is a serious obstacle—how do we actually accomplish the removal of the profit incentive?

The solution seems clear: redirect payments for medical services directly to the doctors and health professionals who actually provide the care. In other words, rather than having payments submitted through an administrative bureaucracy and going into the pockets of those "managing" the HMO, employ a small staff to record payments and distribute money based on fees for services given less a much lower overhead cost. Subsequently, without the middlemen, physicians and medical staff will be paid appropriately and patients will win as their cost will be lower.

So, let's get to work.

The first step in our efforts to eliminate the bureaucracy must be to encourage and generate the political will that ensures everyone has the right to access good health care. This is a political, but necessary, statement because during the birth of our country the idea that all Americans have the right to affordable health care was not included in our Constitution. Most of our government supported medical programs were created subsequent to the administration of Franklin D. Roosevelt.

During recent discussions among the candidates for the presidency of the United States, it appears that Bernie Sanders is on the right track. To quote one of his recent statements, "…every man, woman and child in our country should be able to access the health care they need regardless of their income. We must create a national health care system that provides quality health care for all." Sanders suggests, as do we, that the only long-term solution to our health care crisis is a single-payer national health care program.

The establishment of the Medicare and Medicaid programs was a step in the right direction but the inadequate funding, the absence of Congressional support, and the inadequately designed Affordable Health Care Act will exacerbate the problem by shifting the burden to the states and private insurance companies.

The possible solutions all appear impossible to achieve. Any solution would have to include on-going education for all citizens who will, after all, be patients at some point. That education would focus on preventive health, proper diet and hygiene, quality of life *vis a vis* lifelong medical care and, particularly, what end of life choices should be about. With the abundance of social media, there is no reason that this information cannot be widely and inexpensively disseminated. Unfortunately very little of that information is provided nationwide on a regular basis and, in too many cases, families and individuals avoid discussing these all important issues until the end of life arrives and it is too late to consider how to keep an ailing relative comfortable at home or how to just say, "no" to heroic treatment measures.

As much as many rail against government oversight, we need new laws to require the implementation of the solutions we propose. We need laws to restrict profit-making corporations and institutions from engaging in providing health care; new laws to restrict drug companies and diagnostic hardware manufacturers from driving up the cost of health care while diminishing the diagnostic input of physicians; new laws to restrict physicians and their incorporated organizations from pocketing large amounts of cash gleaned from circuitous methods of multiple billing for the same service; and finally by establishing a realistic tax system to ensure that health care is paid for with specifically designated tax-generated federal dollars rather than by money borrowed from other programs or no money at all.

There are significant challenges to revamping our health care system that are rarely discussed and have been the unspoken rationale for the inaction of Congress. If we are to completely overhaul our health care system, how do we dismantle the current health insurance system? How will the hundreds of thousands of insurance company employees be redirected to other jobs. What will occupy the millions of square feet of office space currently occupied by the health insurance industry? How do we disinvest from the hundreds of profit making drug and medical appliance companies and hospital holding companies without creating national financial chaos? These are the questions that will take the best and brightest thinkers to solve and a citizenry that acknowledges the crisis at hand and indicate a willingness to fix it.

The statements made by Mr. Sanders may point us in the right direction, but there must be real action from the legal system and the government that can only be generated by citizen action if we are to solve our current and future health care crisis.

CHAPTER 13

Transform Hospitals into 21st Century Facilities That Serve Their Communities

The process of re-establishing the original non-profit hospital structure funded by city, county and state tax revenues and philanthropic patrons, could be done simply by looking at the old record books from a few decades ago, then adding the present-day dollar amounts needed to insure that the hospital has the newest technology and well-trained medical staff available for all patients.

To accomplish this may require that hospitals and patients and their families accept the fact that huge expenses for end of life care would have to be replaced with proper nursing or hospice care at home.

CHAPTER 14

The Medical School Curriculum— How to Ensure that Patient Care is Not Synonymous with For-profit Industry

For medical schools to remind students that they are attending medical school to become doctors, not to become rich business people, will be a challenging task in a country that has taught its young people that industrious behavior is rewarded financially while less-industrious individuals should suffer.

Obviously, just being accepted into medical school provides confirmation to the aspiring physician that they are indeed among the intelligent, industrious segment of society. In addition, they have spent a great deal of their parents' money to get there, and they will have to spend considerably more resources to complete their education. There must be a system to enable the graduate doctor to get this money back—with interest.

To be fair, having the society that requires and receives medical care pay the tuition of their care givers from tax revenue seems reasonable. That said, during the training of our physicians how do we ignite a sense of purpose and restore the sense of fulfillment and satisfaction that comes from providing expert care to ones fellow human beings?

CHAPTER 15

How Can Citizen-Patients and Their Families Help to Reinvent Medical Care?

We are witnessing a medical crisis in the making. The main thing we can all do—physicians, patients, concerned citizens—is to be sure we do not stand by silently and watch. We must make our voices heard by those who we have elected to look out for our society.

The authors of this book have studied health care systems in many parts of the world. We have calculated the costs to individuals where health care is looked upon as a social responsibility and a right for all (such as in the Scandinavian countries), and we have looked at the costs to the third world countries where health care is a distant gift, and we have examined the costs to rich countries like the United States where a third of the population has inadequate nutrition and no health care because the system of capitalism demands that the rich are to be rewarded and that the poor must be lazy and be penalized as a result. We have determined that responsible voices must be heard including ours.

The first step in any educational process is to define the problem or question we need to learn about. This is a considerable challenge for health care system because those involved in delivering care are generally considered (and often consider themselves) to be highly informed and able to provide patients, medical association members, or political voting base with the best possible service.

We are taking a risk here by pointing out that, in spite of most physicians being dedicated to truthful and informed service, there are major deficiencies in the information-and-delivery-of-service chain.

Here we will provide sufficient examples to provoke us all to accept the need for a new mindset about health care delivery while not being too defensive about past failures.

Busy primary care physicians face a serious information transfer problem. This information gap results from several factors: often, many years have elapsed between medical school education and the present; annual medical conferences provide only a snapshot of current medical breakthroughs and are inadequate for keeping physicians up-to-date with the abundance of information needed to perform at the highest level; and there is little time for attendance at continuing education courses. A physician's failure to be "up-to-date" is due partly to the fact that the medical school curriculum of years ago did not cover issues important to quality of life today; and annual conferences focus predominantly on new technologies, not on the changing needs and attitudes about health management. As Burton and Hall pointed out in their book, the field of geriatrics did not even exist when they were in medical school. Much of the important information they conveyed to their readers was a result of many years of dedicated experience.

As part of a new and, we believe, necessary mindset we would like to remind physicians and government officials of their duty to consider their new and important role in the health care industry. Here we are employing the commonly used phrase "health care industry" because this is the reality and the challenge each of us must face—health care has become an industry. This fact has good and bad features and we must spend the time to tease out the good, discard the bad, and devise a new method of delivering health care.

Here we ask the question and present a major premise of this book: Is health care really an industry like any other or is it an absolute need and right for all? We believe the concept of health care as "industry" must be removed and be replaced by the belief that health care is an absolute need and an absolute right.

Once we remove the word "industry" what exactly is universal health care? We believe that universal health care is about being interested in adequate nutrition for all people, supporting human dignity, and assuring that every human being is able to maintain a reasonably functional, satisfying existence throughout their lifetime.

For some reason society has decided that individual physicians should fulfill the challenge of providing universal health care—a totally unrealistic premise. At present, the physician is dependent on receiving timely medical information from organizations like pharmaceutical companies or physician practice associations that are focused on their own bottom lines rather than on patients' inability to keep up with the escalating costs of health care. And so it falls upon the physician to make up for the inadequate funding for patient health care needs and decide the future of his patient! This is the political reality and the political impossibility.

Doctors have become victims of the health care industry just as have the patients. There is only one way to repair this mess—we must develop a system that allows physicians to re-educate themselves about how to help the patient so in need of medical, social, and quality of life care.

We believe that every physician must become an activist and an advocate for his or her patients. The physician must enter the fray and be on the front line of revising health care insurance and pension plans. The physician must be an activist that requires a reasonable payment for the services they provide. Then those same physicians must stand before the politicians and insist that the elder generation they represent will not tolerate further exclusion from the social-community process.

A major task for each person participating in the current health care environment is to take responsibility for telling their physician that they are aware that they are likely to be misinformed by the pharmaceutically-driven media, the United States Food and Drug Administration (FDA), and the academic medical community and then support—even insist on—change.

CHAPTER 16

The Future of Health Care Requires Our Immediate Attention

We have considered the many problems facing our health care system and we find four issues to be the most significant.

Problem 1. The current medical education system is turning doctors into debtors. A new doctor, on the day of graduation from medical school, may have a total educational debt between $200,000 and $500,000. As a result, earnings become the most important concern—many doctors literally cannot afford to make their patients' well-being their primary concern.

Problem 2. Instead of being compassionate listeners, relevant information gatherers, and advocates for their patients, medical doctors have become pill pushers and new tests recommenders. In order to get the best deal for him- or her-self, and pay the office rental and the nursing staff, the doctor orders as rapidly as possible an endless array of tests for which the patient is billed. The amount of money paid for the doctor to actually converse with his patient is miniscule compared to the amount received for each test ordered, procedure done or pill prescribed. When the doctor enters the room he may briefly greet the patient before attaching himself to the computer and begin the ordering process. He may glance at some test results on the screen and may even ask a few questions of the patient, but then more tests or procedures will be ordered and a follow-up appointment scheduled. The obvious missing component is the time needed by talking to the patient to become the translator and advocate he has been trained to be.

When one of the authors of this book was an administrator of a neurology practice, she was told that the doctors were expected to spend seven minutes with each patient—"Seven Minutes?" she asked. She responded by telling the bureaucrats that the average neurology patient might take seven minutes just to sit down. Needless to say, the department could not comply with the seven minute rule so their budget allocation was reduced.

Problem 3. By taking advantage of the debtor status of physicians, the pharmaceutical companies found ways to "pay" physicians to recruit patients for clinical trials and to prescribe the newest most expensive medications. As a result, physicians became spokespersons for the industry rather than assessing what was the best course for their patients.

Problem 4. Doctors learned that they had to take a defensive position in the practice of their profession in order to contend with frivolous malpractice suits, class action suits that recruit patients via television ads, and the desire on the part of insurance companies to make financial settlements simply to avoid the time and expense of a court appearance. Thus, playing defense has become a justification for needless tests, MRIs, CT scans, and, most recently, 3-D imaging. Both the potential for litigation and the costs of the tests drive up the medical costs to the patient. Why bother to get to know your patient when an unnecessary test can solve all kinds of problems for the doctor?

The major question that has arisen over the past 20 years is, how do we fix the mess that has been created? What follows are some obvious, but difficult, solutions.

Solution 1. The cost of medical school and medical training must be reduced, or paid for by means other than the graduating physician. Medical school tuition debt must be paid by a system that allows the recent graduate to provide care to all patients in exchange for being debt free. One approach would be to make sure those funds are provided by the wealthiest philanthropists in our society. These people, we all know who they are, rather than providing bed nets in Africa, or polio vaccines in Asia, should be willing to pick up the tab for the suffering American poor. Without the anxiety caused by crushing debt, physicians could once again put their patient first. It is reasonable to expect that compassion and scientific curiosity would return to the world of medicine.

Solution 2. Pharmaceutical companies, laboratories, and for-profit imaging facilities should be banded, by law, from offering physicians financial gain by ordering multiple tests and medications. The examples of this process have been described in this book, but they include, bone density measurements on a population where 90% of women will show low levels, but they do not have more fractures— they still get repeated measurements and drugs. They include PAP smears and pregnancy tests for those over 80 years of age. They include falsely elevating the number of people diagnosed with type 2 diabetes, Alzheimers, and Parkinson's—as these are primarily clinical diagnoses that cannot be verified—then providing lifetime prescriptions and follow-up medical visits to avoid the numerous side effects of the drugs given. Yes, control of this industry must be a part of the solution.

Solution 3. It must be made illegal for pharmaceutical companies or medical equipment companies to provide and financial incentives to hospital administrators, CEOs or Boards of Directors to purchase costly, often redundant, imaging equipment.

Solution 4. The idea that hospitals are better run when they are for-profit must end. The hospital CEOs, COOs, vice presidents, and other administrators make millions of dollars, while the nursing staff and support staff, that includes transport workers and housekeepers, has been drastically slashed and those who remain receive woefully inadequate compensation. This upside-down pyramid must be corrected if patients are to be well cared for.

SUMMARY

There is a Crisis in Health Care—Call Your Doctor!

This book has tried to outline where we now stand on the issues of proper patient care. The authors have not wished simply to return to the glorious past but to identify what has happened to the old family doctor tradition and to find a way to salvage the part of that tradition that can insure that the wonderful activity of attention to patient first and foremost can be preserved. It will be a difficult task as the pressures are tremendous in the other direction. But it is possible to reverse inappropriate and possibly illegal pharmaceutical company advertising and physician payments, to find a way for government funding of education so that young doctors do not feel bound to financial gain rather than social responsibility, and to set up a structure of health care delivery that does not require fee-for service hospitals and clinics.

We, as doctors, nurses and medical educators believe it can be done. We also believe the concept of a doctor who is only interested in his or her

patient's well-being has not really died but has been put on hold by false advertising, short term financial gains, and technology—temporarily, we hope.

Help us help your doctor to see what fun and personal fulfillment proper attention to his or her patients can bring. You can do it. Call your doctor!

REFERENCES

Chapter 3

Jones, T.C and Cotton, J. Aging Aggressively: How to Avoid the US Health-Care Crisis. Balboa Press, 2013, 45-52

Jankovic, J. Parkinson`s Disease: Clinical Features and Diagnosis. J Neurology, Neurosurgery, and Psychiatry. 79: (4) 2007, 368-376

Hansen, R.W. and Higgs, R. Hazardous to Your Health? FDA Regulation of Health Care Products. The Independent Institute, 1995, 13-27.

Angell, M. The Pharmaceutical Industry—To WhomIs It Accountable? New England J Med 2000, 1902-1904.

Chapter 4

Goldacre, B. Bad Science, Forth Estate, London, 2008; 256-27

Szmukler, G. Risk Assessment. "Numbers" and "Va lues". Psych Bull; 2003, 27: 205-207 87

Goldacre, B. Bad Pharma, Forth Estate, London, 2012; 173-224

Bardy, AH. Bias in Reporting Clinical Trials. Brit J Clinical Pharmaco. 1998; 46: 147-150

Chapter 6

Jones, T.C. From Outside Looking Further Out. Balboa Press. 2014, 65-70

Hazzard, W.R. 2001: An American health care odyssey. Ann Int Med 1997; 126: 658-65

Hall, M.A. and Berenson, R.A. Ethical practice in managed care: A dose of realism. Ann Int Med 1998; 128: 395-402

Davidoff, F. Medicine and commerce. 1: Is managed care a "monstrous hybrid"? Ann Int Med 1998; 128: 496-499

Barondess, J. Care of the medical ethos: Reflections on social Darwinism, race hygiene, and the holocaust. Ann Int Med 1998; 129: 891-898

Relman, A. The economic future of health. New Eng J Med 1998; 338: 1855-1856

Andrulis, D.P. Access to care is the centerpiece in the elimination of socioeconomic disparities in health. Ann Int Med 1998; 129:412-416

Council on Ethical and Judicial Affairs, American Medical Association. Ethical issues in managed care. New Eng J Med 1995; 273: 330-335

American College of Physicians. Universal coverage: Renewing the call to action. American College of Physicians, Philadelphia, 1996

Gundersen, L. Number of uninsured continues to rise. Ann Int Med 1998; 129: 513-515

Chapter 10

Mintzes, B. Direct to Consumer Advertising is Medicalising Normal Human Experience. Brit Med J 324: 908-911, 2002

Editorial Board, Turn the Volume Down on Drug Ads. The New York Times, Nov. 27, 2015

Chapter 11

Smith, R. In Search of Non-Diseases. Brit Med J 324: 883-885, 2002

Stone, J. What Should we Say to Patients withSy mptoms Unexplained by Disease? The "Number Needed to Offend." Brit Med J 325:1449-1450, 2002

Chapter 12

Sanders, B. A Single Payment System Like Medicare is the Cure for America's Ailing Health Care. theguardian. com, Sept. 30, 2013

ABOUT THE AUTHORS

Thomas C. Jones, M.D. was born and raised in Medina, Ohio; graduated from Allegheny College and, to follow in his father's footsteps, attended and graduated from the Case Western Reserve Medical School in 1962. Dr. Jones completed his internship and residency training and a one-year fellowship in infectious diseases at Cornell University Medical College-The New York Hospital in 1967. He served as captain in the United States Air Force stationed at Clark Air Base in the Philippines 1967 to 1969. He did cell research at The Rockefeller University and completed an infectious diseases fellowship in 1972. He was professor of infectious diseases and public health and chief of the Division International Medicine at Cornell University Medical College until 1985. Currently, he is emeritus adjunct professor of medicine and public health at Weill-Cornell Medical College.

Dr. Jones served as medical expert and then head of the Division of Infectious Diseases, Dermatology and Asthma at Sandoz Pharmaceutical Ag., Basle,

Switzerland (1985–1995) following which he was head of Clinical Research Associates in Basle (1995–2005).

Jones wrote *The Medical Care of Refugees* (Oxford University Press, New York, 1987) and has published over 200 research articles in the medical literature. He was the first editor of the *Brazilian Journal of Infectious Diseases* (1996–2001).

His principal philosophy about health care is described in this book and includes the need for transparency in all aspects of health care, universal attention to basic needs of nutrition and health everywhere in the world, and a careful understanding of the need for quality of life care at the end of life, not heroic measures to extend life.

Betsy M. Chalfin, M.Ed. graduated from Northwestern University with a BA in History and received her M.Ed. in special education from the University of Illinois, Chicago. She was program coordinator for the Division of International Medicine at Cornell University Medical School and went on to serve as the medical program director for the International Rescue Committee in 1984. In 1991, she became director of residency recruitment and academic administrator in the Department of Neurology at the Mount Sinai School of Medicine; later she became administrator for the Department of Neurology at the Beth Israel Medical Center. Ms. Chalfin was copy editor for the *Brazilian Journal of Infectious Diseases* 1996–2001. She has continued to follow the current state of health care, supports local community health programs in North Carolina, and works for political candidates who advocate for a government-provided single-payer health care plan for all.

Printed in the United States
By Bookmasters